Risque Beauty

Beauty Secrets of History's Most Notorious Courtesans

Edited by
Daniela Turudich

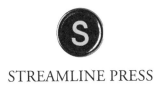

STREAMLINE PRESS

For my family.

Published by Streamline Press
www.StreamlinePressShop.com

First Edition
ISBN: 1-930064-18-7

Distributed to the book trade by IPG, Chicago.

Other fine books from Streamline Press are available online at: www.StreamlinePressShop.com or from your local bookstore.

Contents

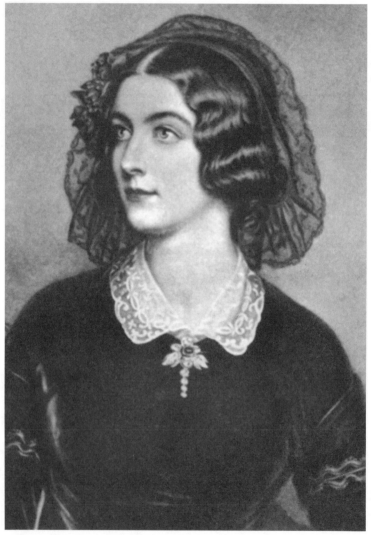

Editor's Note

Dear reader, welcome to our collection of hidden beauty secrets from some of history's most famous courtesan's. This collection is the first of its kind.

The recipes, tips, instructions, and secrets are from period sources and are historically accurate and authentic in nature. We have taken great pains to remove recipes and secrets that were obviously dangerous (those containing lead and mercury), and have included those which may be easily replicated at home. If you are unsure about any of the recipes or ingredients, please seek advice before attempting.

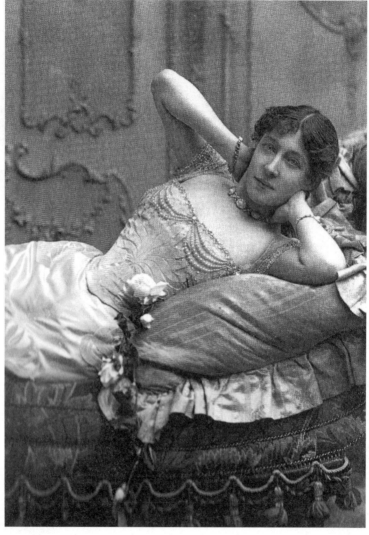

Every woman has a story and every courtesan has a scandalous one. Captured in these pages are the histories and beauty secrets of some of the most notorious courtesans the world has ever known.

What are Courtesans?

Courtesan, noun: a kept woman or prostitute associating with noblemen or men of wealth.

Also known as ...
Demimondaine (French)
Grande Horizontales
Cortigiana (Italian)

Courtesans were kept women who created lives for themselves by accepting gifts and favors from admirers in exchange for companionship. Were they prostitutes? Yes, and their "clients" were noblemen and kings. Courtesans dressed like royalty and most were highly educated, cultured and witty.

Most did not intend to become a courtesan, but fell into their careers as a solution to various life circumstances.

These women were independent and clever. They knew how to attract and retain admirers. Although renowned for being beautiful, many of the world's most famous courtesans weren't overly attractive. In fact, some were classically… ugly. However, they were intelligent enough to make themselves seem intriguing and desirable sometimes by sheer force of their character alone. That's right girls, personality. That and a little public relations to build their image in the minds of their lovers and of the public – worked magic to seal their fates in our collective history.

"They created for themselves a situation almost equivalent to that of a man ..free in behavior and conversation, attaining "the rarest intellectual liberty".
~ Simone de Beauvoir

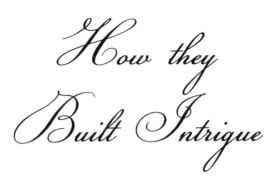

How they Built Intrigue

Fiercely Independent

These women carved out a life during times when marriage had little to do with romance. Marriage was a contractual obligation, and very few were entered into with a foundation built of love. For many women, the life of a courtesan was more appealing than being bound in matrimony to a man they may have despised. After all, as courtesans they could choose their lovers.

This fierce independence also helped build intrigue in their dealings with lovers. Their lovers could have them for a night, but never for a lifetime. These were women that understood that men, even kings, loved the art of the chase. They understood that part of what made them intriguing was the idea and illusion that they could never be "tamed." They were wild, hidden and fun. They were all of the things that regular housewives were not allowed to be.

Intellect and Wit
"Beauty fades, but dumb is forever." Judith Scheindlin

"Wit in women is a jewel, which, unlike all others, borrows lustre from its setting, rather than bestows it; since nothing is so easy as to fancy a very beautiful woman extremely witty." Colton

There is an ongoing myth that in order to have been a famous courtesan, the women must have been the most beautiful and attractive of their time. This is most often not the case. The most famous and influential women, were often not the prettiest, but offered something more. The courtesans who focused on their personal beauty to retain the attraction of their lovers inadvertently had the shortest career. Beauty fades, and many beautiful but boring women were quickly replaced and forgotten when a younger, fresher face came to court. However, the courtesans that skillfully mixed beauty with intellect and wit enjoyed decades of attention. They were bright, funny, and smart and typically held the greatest sway for the longest lengths of time with the highest levels of nobility.

Public Relations and Advertising

How does a courtesan become well known and famous, attracting admirers from all over the world? Public relations and advertising. Back then, it was not so different than it is today. To become well known and attract wealthy patrons, courtesans needed to "manage" their public image. They would dress in extraordinarily fine clothing that was a bit risqué and make sure they were seen about town. They would make sure that stories were written about them and that people gossiped about them. They would hold salons and dinner parties with the most respected, intellectual, and famous guests they could assemble. They would have feuds among themselves and commission or sit for portraits of themselves. They would go to extravagancies – just to ensure that they were never confused for being dull, boring, or domesticated – the antithesis of what a courtesan offered to her patrons and admirers. For above all, the world of the courtesan was a dream, a hallucination, one that a patron could enter and exit at will without affecting "real life."

A successful courtesan was a master of psychological and image manipulation.

The Ladies

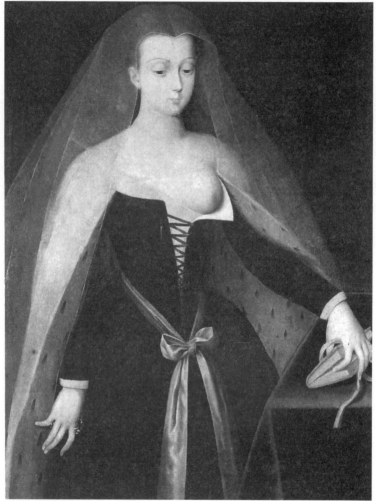

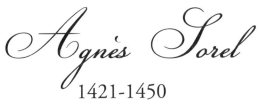

Agnès Sorel
1421-1450
Born: Fromenteau in Touraine, France

Who Was Agnès?

Agnès is considered the "first official royal mistress" in France. She was mistress to King Charles VII of France and is beloved by the French people still to this day. Her influence over the King is a tale of legend. She is credited with pulling the King out of a protracted depression and with helping turn him from a weak and timid figurehead to a strong and decisive King. She was not a fragile woman. She would accompanied the king by horseback on hunting parties and hated flattery and double faced dealings.

The King's reign during the time of Agnès, turned to be his most prosperous. Agnès died an early death at the age of 28 and speculation is that she was murdered due to her influence over the King. However, later autopsies showed she may have died due to cosmetic mercury poisoning. She is a beloved figure in French history.

The Beauty and Intrigue of Agnès

Agnès was extraordinarily beautiful and extremely intelligent. Often referred to as the Dame de beauté, Agnès had golden hair and light blue eyes. Agnès was known for extravagant displays. She wore trains a third longer than any princess and had a much grander wardrobe. She designed the clothes herself and often wore low cut gowns that exposed her shoulders as well as her bosom. Gowns were of silk or satin with fur lining. She would display one or both of her breasts while at court, common fashion during the time period. She is reported as having the most beautiful breasts in 15th Century Europe. Under everything Agnes had another surprise for the King. Instead of common undergarments of wool, they were dainty and made of linen. Agnès often wore hair in ringlets, or curls simply tied with a bow at the nape of neck. Clothing and hair were decidedly sensual and non-restrictive.

Perfumed Clothing

Agnès knew the power of seduction and scent. She loved ambergris which had a fragrance much like musk and had her cloaks soaked in the scent. Although ambergris is not readily available these days, a similar effect can be achieved with musk perfume or any other perfume you prefer. Simply soak a swatch of fabric in the scent and sew the fabric swatch into the lining of clothing or your brassiere. As your body heats up it will activate the perfume and provide a lingering scent.

Perfumed Skin

Agnès is thought to have used powder Iris roots as body scent. Iris roots (commonly now referred to as orris root) were ground into a powder that gave off a soft violet scent. The powder was used as an aphrodisiac. Orris root also reduces the appearance of wrinkles by hydrating and increasing skin elasticity. Orris root powder can be procured today and can be lightly dusted on the body after a bath.

Honey Facial Preparations

Agnès is thought to have used honey facial preparations as a beauty treatment.

Egg and Honey Mask

Beat the white of one egg and mix in 1 tablespoon of honey. Apply to the skin. Leave on for fifteen minutes. Rinse off with tepid water.

Honey Mask

Smear honey on the face and leave on for 15 minutes. Wash off with tepid water.

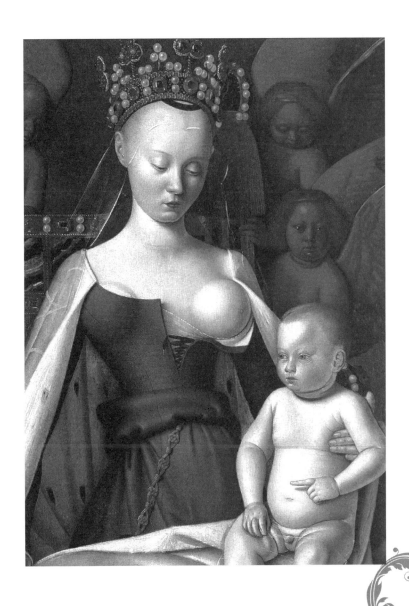

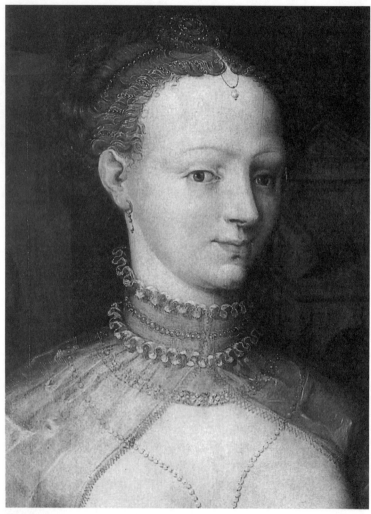

Diane de Poitiers

1499–1566

Born: Château de Saint-Vallier, in the town of Saint-Vallier, Drôme, in the Rhône-Alpes region of France.

Who Was Diane?

Diane was the official mistress of King Henry II of France. Her career as a mistress began after the death of her husband who was noted as being one of the ugliest men of his time. Upon her husband's death, Diane attended a tournament at which time the Duke of Orleans (Henry, one of the King's sons) broke a lance in her honor. She was 31 years old and he was 14. From that moment on he was never away from her. Until his father's death, in 1547, it may be said that no one knew what Henry was, except Diane de Poitiers. By the time Henry became King, he was already married to Catherine de Medici. Diane was 48 and he was 31. He lent upon her absolutely; even in public, he never made a decision without first glancing at her for counsel. Diane possessed a sharp intellect and was so politically astute that King Henry II trusted her to write many of his official letters, and even to sign them jointly with the one name HenriDiane.

Diane surrounded the King with loveliness wherever he turned. This was genius since he was naturally morose. She amused as well as dazzled him. She was not content with making him fall in love — she plunged him in "a perpetual state of ecstasy." Her expenditure was enormous, but the Royal Treasury paid; and she had other ways and means as well. She levied taxes on everything she could in her own domain.

In 1559 the King became injured in a tournament and died 11 days later. Shortly thereafter, Catherine de Medici took her revenge on Diane and banished her from court.

The Beauty and Intrigue of Diane

Diane's beauty was a very debatable question. She had a brilliant complexion and her bath and morning ritual regimen enhanced it; for the rest, the distinctive character of her aspect was health, not loveliness. This lady was not quite pretty, but she was divinely fresh.

Diane's Infamous Ice-Water Bath & Morning Ritual

Diane would wake everyday at 5am and take an ice cold bath. This was rare for the time when daily bathing and personal cleanliness was rare.

After the legendary "tub," Diane would hunt on horseback for two or three hours. She believed that "an hour's exercise in the morning air before the morning dew had left" was key to maintaining her freshness.

Diane's Spring Water / Rain Water Facial Rinse

Diane washed her face with spring water. Spring water contains trace amounts of natural minerals that help calm and soothe sensitive skin.

Diane's Milk Bath

Milk would be added to the bath when extra soothing and moisturizing was intended. Milk is purported to have anti-oxidant and anti-aging properties thereby slowing down the aging process. Used throughout history as a beauty regime.

Add one to two cups of fresh or powdered milk to your bath water.

Diane's Complexion Recipe

White turpentine, lily roots, honey, eggs, egg shells, camphor, mixed up and boiled in the inside of a pigeon. *Not to be tried at home.*

Diane's Elixir of Youth

In 2009, French experts examined the remains of Diane de Poitiers and found extraordinary levels of gold in her hair. It is believed that she regularly drank an elixir made with gold that she believed would preserve her youth. This "drinkable gold" may have killed her. *Not to be tried at home.*

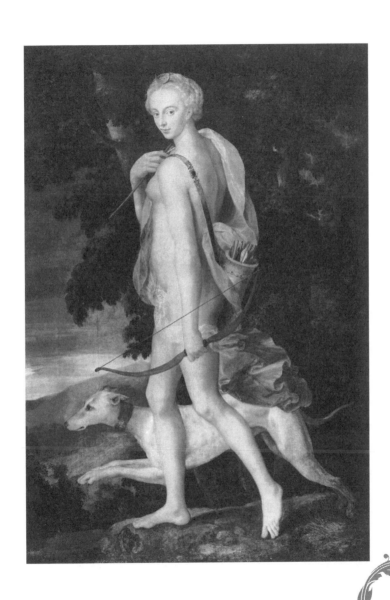

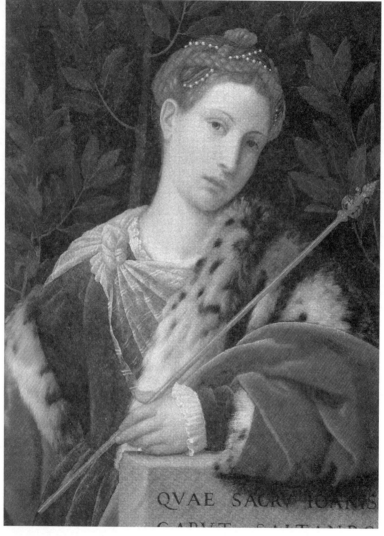

QVAE SACRV IOANIS

"She is not as you say, beautiful; but she is highly gifted in talent and wit."

Tullia d'Aragona

1510–1556
Born: Rome, Italy

Who Was Tullia?

Tullia was the daughter of a courtesan. Her mother was lauded as one of the most famous beauties of her day. The identity of Tullia's father is unknown but is widely thought to have been Cardinal Luigi d'Aragona. Tullia was a child prodigy from a young age and was not known for her beauty, the way her mother was. Instead, Tullia amazed and entertained powerful men with her sharp tongue and wit. She was educated and cultured and her literary abilities made her a successful writer and infamous as a courtesan. The house of La Tullia was frequented by the "best of society."

The Beauty and Intrigue of Tullia

Tullia had yellow hair and remarkably large and bright eyes. Her eyes would disarm those that came near her.

Tullia's Color for Beauty

Tullia always loved the color red, both for itself and because it made her complexion appear less florid by contrast. Know your coloring and use it to downplay flaws and to bring out your best assets.

For a Naturally Red Face

Take four ounces the kernels (soft pit inside of the fruit stone) of peaches and two ounces gourd seeds and make them into an oil. Apply this to the face.

To Take Red Pimples out of Fair Faces

Mix rock salt with white of one egg. Boil over heat while stirring until it thickens. Apply to red spots every day for 3-4 days.

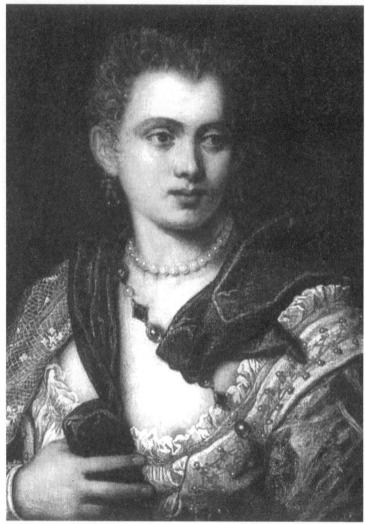

Veronica Franco

1546–1591
Born: Venice, Italy

Who was Veronica?
Veronica was born to a middle class family in Venice and in early life married a doctor. She was highly cultured and spoke several languages. She also sang well and played many musical instruments. She was a published poet and was once the lover to King Henry III of France.

"Even if fate should be completely favorable and kind to a young woman, this is a life that always turns out to be a misery. It's a most wretched thing, contrary to human reason, to subject one's body and labor to a slavery terrifying even to think of. To make oneself prey to so many men, at the risk of being stripped, robbed, even killed, so that one man, one day, may snatch away from you everything you've acquired from many over such a long time, along with so many other dangers of injury and dreadful contagious diseases; to eat with another's mouth, sleep with another's eyes, move accordingly to another's will, obviously rushing towards the shipwreck of your mind and your body – what greater misery?

What wealth, what luxuries, what delights can outweigh all this? Believe me, among all the world's calamities, this is the worst."
~ Veronica Franco

The Intrigue of Venetian Courtesans
It was custom for a Venetian prostitute to have 6 or 7 gentlemen as clients at a time. Each was allowed to sup and sleep with her one night a week leaving her days free. They paid her a monthly fee/retainer, but she was always free to accept someone new passing through and rearrange an evening visit with one of her regulars. Venetian courtesans loved display and extravagance. They would travel in red lit gondolas in their low-necked dresses and curly hair and wigs. They had under-linens and bedclothes that were lined with silver and gold thread. They took better care of themselves and bathed more frequently than the great ladies of Venice.

It was the special duty of the waiting maids to take extra pains to make their mistresses attractive: using cosmetics, dressing the hair in ringlets, rolls and tresses, loading the arms up with bracelets, the rings with fingers, the ears with pendants, dressing them in the most sumptuous clothing. When this elaborate toilette was finished, each courtesan would send pages out with notes, full of phrases of affection to their lovers. While awaiting their lovers, they would seat themselves at the window or balcony surrounded by small pets.

Venetian Courtesan's Aphrodisiac Bath Water

The water for the bath was scented with aromatic herbs that gave a delicate scent to the body. When the courtesan left her bath she was carefully dried by her maidens, her body perfumed, and her nails polished.

Add a 8-10 drops of cedar wood oil to warm bath water. The scent of cedar was thought to be an aphrodisiac.

Rosemary Water Facial Rinse

Take a handful of rosemary flowers and boil them in white wine. When cool, use as a facial wash.

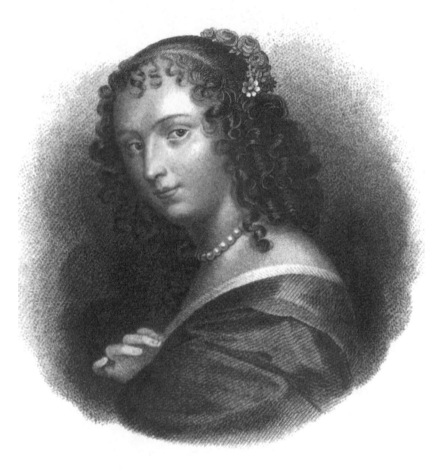

*"She was a problem even for her own time. One must
be a philosopher to appreciate her fully. No writer
could render such a character"*

Ninon de l'Enclos

1615–1705
Born: Paris, France
Birth Name: Anne de l'Enclos

"I saw, as soon as I began to reflect, that our sex has been burdened with all that is frivolous, and that men have reserved to themselves the right to the essential things and qualities. From that moment, I resolved to make myself a man."
~Ninon

"I think I may love you for three months, and that's an eternity for me."
~Ninon

Who was Ninon?
Ninon was an infamous courtesan. She had what the French call esprit (wit; lively intelligence). Saint-Simon noted Ninon made friends among the great in every walk of life, had wit and intelligence enough to keep them, and, what is more, to keep them friendly with one another.

"Ninon always had crowds of adorers but never more than one lover at a time, and when she tired of the present occupier, she said so frankly and took another. Yet such was the authority of this wanton, that no man dared fall out with his successful rival; he was only too happy to be allowed to visit as a familiar friend."

Her own talk was natural always, witty often ; literature and art were her favorite topics — Moliere used to consult her, "for she has the keenest sense of the absurd of any one I know"; and she was, besides, a brilliant mimic. She had done just what she liked — and had never been afraid.

From an early age her father trained her to understand three classes of adorers:
1. the 'payers' whom she cared nothing for and only made use of till she could do without them
2. the 'martyrs'
3. the ' favorites'

On his death-bed he enforced it further. "Be scrupulous" he said, "only in the choice of your pleasures — never mind about the number."

The Intrigue of Ninon

There is an old Parisian legend about Ninon. The legend says that she had made a pact with the devil in exchange for eternal beauty. Her name became synonymous with beauty and a multitude of beauty products sprang up utilizing her name. Ninon also had conversational wit and spirit. "Her mind was more attractive than her face," The truth is, of course, that she had fascination — that self-made beauty, as it were, which lives forever, as her legend lives, which goes beyond mere facial loveliness, even when they go together. A frank and tender, touching face, an arresting voice, a dazzling skin, a faultless figure, grace in every movement....

Some of Ninon's personal beauty secrets included:
- Never drinking wine, she never drank anything but water
- Never wearing rouge, even though was very popular
- Using reddish-brown Marechal powder in her hair
- Adding perfume to gloves, fans, perfumes
- Wearing a kissing patch like a tiny star in one of the dimples at the corner of her mouth

Ninon's Lemon & Salt Face Scrub

Mix the juice of one lemon with table salt. Apply to the skin and rinse.

Ninon's Asses Milk (Donkey Milk) Bath

Asses milk baths are an age old anti-aging secret. It is said that even Cleopatra bathed in Asses milk.
Add one to two cups liquid or powdered donkey milk to your bath water.

Ninon's Alkali Bath

Liked her baths with a pinch of alkali (baking soda). Baking soda baths are detoxifying and used to sooth and treat skin disorders. Add one half to one cup of baking soda to your bath water.

Crème de l'enclose (famous Parisian cosmetic)

½ pint whole milk
¼ ounce lemon juice
¼ ounce white brandy
Boil all together and skim off scum. Use it night and
morning.

Pomade de Ninon

4 ounces oil of sweet almonds
3 ounces washed lard
3 ounces juice of house leek

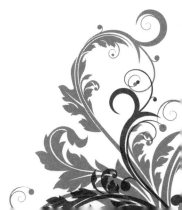

Kissing Patch

Kissing patches were made to accentuate features and to cover up facial scars and pox caused by caustic cosmetics. Patches were made of black taffeta, velvet, silk, or thin leather and cut into tiny circles, stars, crescents, and hearts. They were stuck to the face using glue made from gum mastic.

Where the patches were located held special meaning for example is worn near the mouth meant boldness. If worn near the eye it meant passion.

Patch Glue

Powdered mastic (gum Arabic) is mixed with water in a 1:6 ratio (i.e. 1 teaspoon of powdered mastic to 6 teaspoons of water). It will produce a gummy substance than can be used as an adhesive for the patch. More or less water may be added to achieve the consistency you desire.

A Marechal Powder Recipe
(Hair Powder)

Marechal (also known as Marechele Powder) was powder that was sprinkled onto the hair to absorb grease and impart a pleasant aroma to unwashed hair. Marechal powder is described as either reddish brown or yellow in coloring. The tint depended on what type of sandalwood was used (yellow or red).

½ pound orris root powder

½ pound sandalwood powder (can be red or yellow)

¼ pound ground rose petal powder

½ pound ground cloves

¼ pound ground cinnamon

¼ dram musk grains

And easier version of this recipe is to simply use ground orris root.

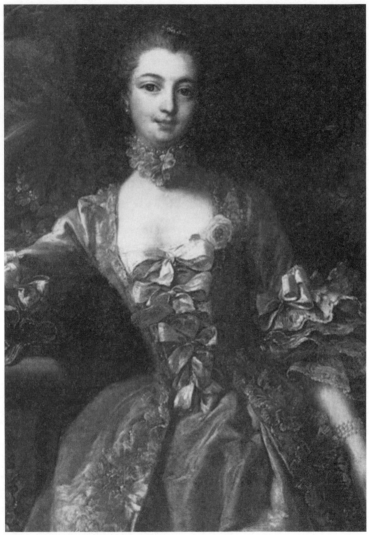

Madame de Pompadour

1721–1764
Born: Paris, France
Birth Name: Jeanne Antoinette Poisson

*Pompadour you embellish
the court....
Now that Louis has returned
May you both enjoy peace
And both keep your conquests
~ Voltaire*

Who Was Madame de Pompadour

Pompadour was the official chief mistress of King Louis XV. She was born in Paris and well educated. She was married at 19 and became involved in the Parisian social circles, hosting her own salon and inviting many philosophers of the time. As she became well known in society, her father-in-law arranged for her to be introduced to the King at a ball. Shortly thereafter, she was installed at Versailles as the King's mistress and it was proclaimed that she and her husband had separated.

Behind the scenes, Pompadour had a considerable amount of influence over the King which won her many enemies at court. She made it a point to have a cordial relationship with the queen, which eased Louis guilt. Pompadour also accompanied him hunting and playing cards. She frequently reminded Louis of her beauty by constantly commissioning paintings of herself.

The Intrigue of Pompadour

Madame de Pompadour was beautiful. She had a small mouth, oval face and was full of fun and spirit. She spent a considerable amount of effort and time into making the King's life fun and joyous. Madame de Pompadour liked to use rouge, patching, pearl powder and musk.

Pompadour's Morning Cucumber Cleanse

It is said that Pompadour used to wipe her face every morning with a soft cloth dipped in cucumber juice.

Pompadour's Olive Oil Skin Treatment

Apply olive oil to the skin and let sit for 10-15 minutes. Wipe off with a cloth dipped in lemon juice, being careful to avoid the eyes.

Pompadour's Skin Nourishment Mask

Fresh carrot juice mixed with a teaspoon of honey and applied to the face as a mask. Rinse with tepid water.

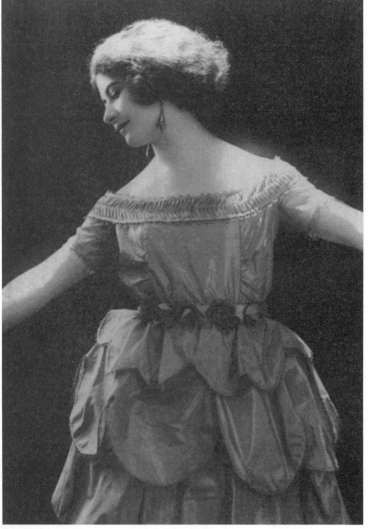

"the prince always found her in the lap of luxury, dazzling in her strange, voluptuous beauty, a beauty which was a little contrived, a little painted, and very artificial."

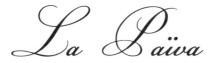

La Païva

1819–1884
Born: Moscow, Russia
Birth Name: Esther Lachmann

Who was La Paiva

Esther Lachmann was one of the most successful 19th
Century French Courtesans. She was born in Moscow to
Jewish Polish decedents. Esther married young and after a
year or two, she left her husband and infant son, and went
to Paris where she took a lover. Once her lover's fortune
was gone, she became a courtesan. Esther was an adept
and shrewd business woman and very ambitious. She was
a notable investor and helped men manage their fortunes.
Although she established herself by her feminine attractions,
she had a masculine toughness. It is recorded that one day,
when she was thrown by a horse, she took a pistol from her
belt and shot the horse with it.

The Intrigue of La Paiva

"She was far from beautiful: her hair was blue-black, her
eyes were slightly protruding, her nose was Mongolian,
while her mouth and chin suggested energy rather than
gentleness.

But if she was unlikely to attract conventional lovers, she possessed a flamboyant exoticism which appealed to more' original men. She had some rare, disturbing quality which commanded the attention."

"White skin, good arms, beautiful shoulders, bare behind down to the hips, the reddish hair under her arms showing each time that she adjusted her shoulder straps; the mouth a straight line cutting across a face all white with rice powder."

La Paiva also took milk baths and lime-flower baths.

Rice Powder Recipe

Rice cosmetic powder is still manufactured today. To make sure you use the finest rice powder possible, pour powder into a stocking, and sift. Rice powder acts much like talc, but is not harmful to the skin the way that talc is.

For a translucent dusting, apply rice powder with a dry cosmetic brush over skin to which has been applied moisturizer or foundation. Loose powder needs something to "stick" to. Dip cosmetic brush into powder, and then tap brush on tissue paper to remove extra powder. Lightly dust over skin.

For more coverage using rice powder, apply powder with a damp sponge (if no foundation) or dry sponge (if a foundation has been applied). Press the powder onto the skin. Buff with a stiff, dry cosmetic brush.

Lime-Flower Herbal Bath (Linden Tea Bath)

A linden tea bath was used to soothe the skin, reduce inflammation, and to keep skin from ageing. Linden tea has natural anti-aging/antioxidant properties.

To make an herbal bath tie up a half cup of linden herb in a muslin bag and fasten it to the spout of the tub so that the hot waters run through it. After the water is drawn, place the bag in the water with you.

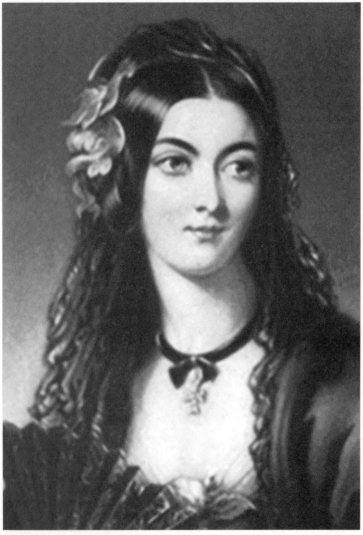

"When you met Lola Montez, her reputation made you automatically think of bedrooms."
~ Aldous Huxley.

Lola Montez

1821-1861
Born: Sligo, Ireland
Birth Name: Eliza Rosanna Gilbert

Who Was Lola?

Lola was an Irish born woman who transformed herself into a "Spanish dancer" and courtesan. She was the mistress of King Ludwig I of Bavaria. As a young girl Eliza was known for her obstinacy and her temper. She was sent from boarding school to boarding school. At one boarding school, an art instructor recalled her as having eyes of "excessive beauty", an "orientally dark" complexion and an air of "haughty ease". At 16, she ran away from home and eloped with a man. Five years later, they separated. It was at that time that her "character" and dancing profession began. She became famous, but more for her beauty and quick temper, than for her dancing skill. She became the mistress of King Ludwig I of Bavaria. After their affair ended, Eliza went back to the stage, eventually landing and staying in America.

The Intrigue of Lola

Lola was intense in both beauty and personality. Dark hair with large blue eyes coupled with dynamic sheer force of character made her unforgettable.

Lola always wore a Byronic collar (collar open wide and the lapels spread open, flat against the chest) which helped the theory, held by many, that she was a daughter of a poet. But her real reason for adopting the style was that she had a lovely neck, and this set it off to the best advantage. Her favorite material was velvet, which she wore to create an erotic effect on men of a certain age. She was insistent, too, that the contours of her figure should be clearly revealed, and in a distinctly provocative fashion.

Lotion for Improving Flexibility

Meant to be rubbed onto the skin in the evening and left on overnight. This lotion was thought to improve muscle and limb flexibility – to allow for, well, all sorts of things.

8 ozs. lanolin
4 ozs. olive oil
3 ozs. white wax
1 grain musk
½ pint white brandy
4 ozs. rose water

Put the fat, oil and wax into an earthen ceramic bowl placed over a pot with water simmering over low heat. Allow fat, oil, and wax to melt together, then pour in other ingredients. Allow to cool. Apply to limbs in the evening and leave on overnight. In the morning wipe down the body with a sponge moistened with cool water.

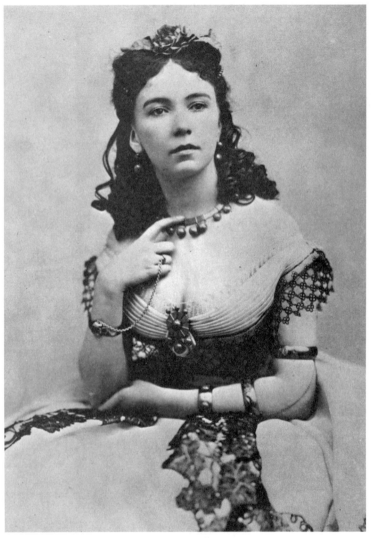

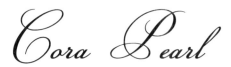

Cora Pearl

1835–1886

Born: London, England
Birth Name: Emma Elizabeth Crouch or
Eliza Emma Crouch

"…I have never deceived anyone, for I have never belonged to anyone. My independence was all my wealth: I have known no other happiness."
~ Cora Pearl

"I have never seized the arm of the first man who came my way. Being the mistress of my own free will, I have kept my independence toward and against all. It was the only way to make men worth my while love me, and to keep myself from being the prey of scamps."
~ Cora Pearl

Who Was Cora?
Cora Pearl was a well known courtesan during the later part of the 19th Century. One day when Cora was 15 years old, she was making her way home and was approached by a 40 year old man. He took her to a bar and filled her full of alcohol. When she woke up, she realized her virginity had been taken.

From that point forward she harbored a deep hatred for men. She never went home and instead took the money the man had left for her and set herself up in lodging. She eventually made her way to Paris and began taking lovers. There, she became famous for pitting lovers against one another.

Cora had many lovers, the most notable being Emperor Napoleon's brother.

The Intrigue of Cora Pearl

Cora believed in spectacle and shock. There are accounts of her dying her hair yellow to match her yellow carriage and dying the fur of her dog blue to match her blue gown. On one occasion, she threw a dinner party to a group of well renowned guests. As her guests assembled around the dinner table, she dared the group "to cut into the next dish" about to be served. The next course was Cora Pearl herself, nude on a platter, sprinkled with parsley, and carried in by four large men.

Cora believed in a few rules when it came to dealing with her lovers:
• Always wear a low cut dress.
• Play hard to get.
• Don't always treat them well, ignore them, etc.

Cora also believed in makeup and used it excessively. She was a fan of face powder tinted with silver or pearl to give her skin a shimmering glow.

Pearl Powder

Pearl Powder was a finely milled powder made of crushed and ground pearl. It was used as a cosmetic powder for the face. It was thought to improve the appearance and to have a purifying effect on the skin. It was widely used as a treatment for acne, a treatment for fading acne scars, and as a cosmetic for highly sensitive skin.

Pearl powder is still available today.

For a translucent dusting, apply pearl powder with a dry cosmetic brush over skin to which has been applied moisturizer or foundation. Loose powder needs something to "stick" to. Dip cosmetic brush into powder, and then tap brush on tissue paper to remove extra powder. Lightly dust over the skin.

For more coverage, apply pearl powder with a damp sponge (if no foundation) or dry sponge (if foundation has been applied). Press the powder onto the skin. Buff with stiff, dry cosmetic brush.

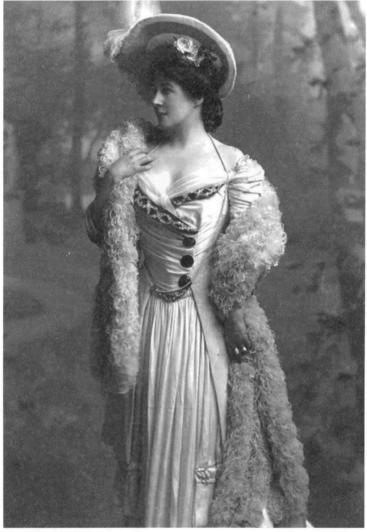

"I resent Mrs. Langtry, she has no right to be intelligent, daring and independent, as well as lovely."
~ George Bernard Shaw

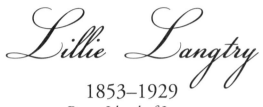

Lillie Langtry

1853–1929

Born: Island of Jersey
Birth Name: Emilie Charlotte Le Breton
Also known as Lily Langtry / Jersey Lil

"Man wears what he pleases, and is guided by only two rules. He dresses for comfort, and to enhance his appearance. Woman is entitled to the same privilege, and if society won't give it to her, she must take it for herself. What looks attractive on someone else might be hideous if I wear it, and vice versa. Every woman is entitled to her independence. It is her right to dress conspicuously or modestly, as she chooses. It is her right to ignore the dictates of fashion and dress in a manner that is most becoming to her own character and personality. In these days when woman is being granted the vote everywhere, we hear she is at last man's equal, but she will not achieve true equality until she breaks the chains of fashion's tyranny and strikes out on her own."
~Lillie Langtry

Who Was Lillie?

Lillie was the only girl in a brood of six children. Growing up around boys she was comfortable around them and understood them. Learning to be feisty from her brothers, she was a handful for her governess and ended being educated by her brothers' tutors.

Lillie married at a young age. She was beautiful and soon attracted the attention of artists, became their muse, and was excitedly introduced into London high society. The excitement over Lillie was palpable and Prince Edward arranged to sit next to her at a dinner while her husband was sat at the other end of the table. The Prince became infatuated with Lillie and she became his mistress. Once the Prince moved on to other conquests, Lillie turned to the stage.

The Intrigue of Lillie

Lillie was the epitome of the 19th century standard of beauty. She was tall, broad hipped and full-bosomed, with a pearly white complexion, and golden brown hair. Lillie once revealed that the secret behind her apparently unchanging fine looks was the habit of daily physical exercise she had developed in her youth.

Lillie also had a gregarious and extroverted personality and was a witty conversationalist.

Lillie Langtry's Secrets of Youth

"Live in color. Think in color -- That Is the secret of eternal youth. Bright thoughts. Bright colors. Bright looks. That's the way to keep Young."

"I avoid sauces, made dishes, and sweets and insist upon simple dishes and not too much, at regular hours.

"The profound secret of keeping young is that I've learned to keep my thoughts young. To a great extent a woman's beauty is measured by her vitality – by her health. Work, sunshine, exercise, water and soap, plain nourishing food, lots of fresh air and a happy, contented spirit – is my working rule for youth, youthful spirit, and youthful looks."

Lillie's Morning Ritual

Lillie would take an icy cold bath in the morning. After the bath, she would do a few exercises – bending and reaching and touching the toes. After stretching, she would take a long walk, keeping up a pretty steady pace for two hours.

Lillie's Evening Rituals

Lillie's evening ritual consisted of a hot bath and full body soap scrub all over, followed by 3-4 minutes of deep breathing. A few more physical exercises, then to bed.

"I sleep with the windows wide open and all the heat turned off. We can't get too much fresh air. I wear very light clothing.

Other Lillie Langtry Advice Tidbits
• Doesn't like to eat alone. Eats very simple dinner.
• Personal impression made by each women in how she carries herself. Always stand straight up, chest must be raised. Never let the chest drop. Stomach in. You should be able to drop a line from the ear, shoulder, hip and instep.

There's a lovely lady in a plain black gown
She isn't very rich, but she's taken all the town
London Society has gone quite silly
Fallen at the feet of the Jersey Lillie
There's the Langtry this and the Langtry that
The Langtry bonnet and the Langtry hat
The Langtry slipper and the Langtry shoe
Langtry purple and a Langtry Blue
The Langtry carriage and Langtry cot
and every woman's hair in the Langtry Knot.
Her profile is certainly Praxetelean;
She makes other Beauties look plain, or plebeian
And readers of fiction observe with surprise
A real live lady with violet eyes.

~ Dorothea Mapelson

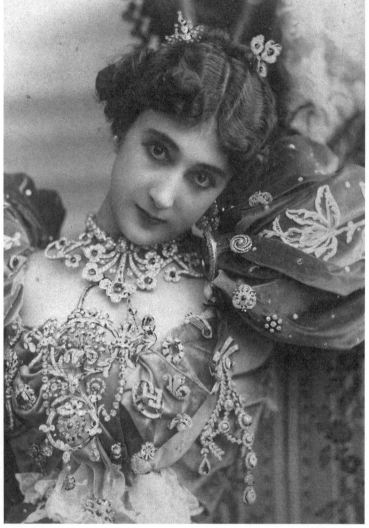

"She danced a little and she was something new, a lot."

La Belle Otero

1868–1965
Born: Valga, Spain
Birth Name: Agustina Otero Iglesias

"Every generation should have the opportunity to pay to see one superlatively lovely women."
~ La Belle Otero

Who was La Belle Otero?

Agustina was born to a very poor family and as a child moved to Santiago de Campostella and found work as a maid. She was raped at 10 years old and as a result was left sterile. At 14 years old she left Santiago de Campostella to start her dancing career. While dancing in Barcelona, she met a benefactor that moved her to Marseille to help promote her dancing career. When she arrived in France, she created the stage character of "La Belle Otero" which was a play on being an Andalusian Gypsy. Her dancing path led her to become a star at the Folies Bergères in Paris and she was considered the best Spanish dancer in France.

La Belle Otero had many lovers and chose them carefully, focusing mainly on Dukes, Princes and Kings.

The Intrigue of La Belle Otero

Agustina was from Spain and naturally exotic for the French public. She wore mantillas, had dark black eyes, dark hair, carmine lips and a voluptuous bosom which was said to inspire the twin cupolas of the Hotel Carlton in Cannes.

Preparation for a Voluptuous Bosom

½ ounce tincture of myrrh
4 ounces pimpernel water
4 ounces elder flower water
1 grain musk
6 ounces rectified spirits of wine
The about preparation very softly rubbed upon the bosom for five or ten minutes, two to three times a day and was used to promote bust growth.

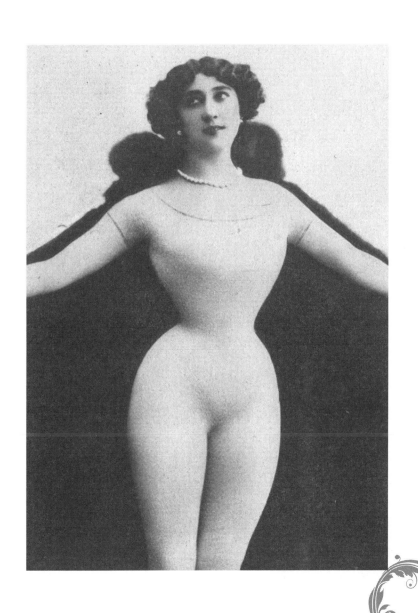

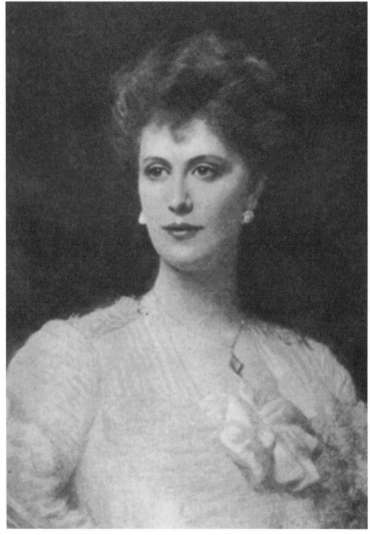

Alice Keppel

1869–1947

Born: Duntreath Castle, Scotland

Who was Alice?

Alice Keppel was a society hostess and married woman who caught the interest of a King.

Along the way she became a well known hostess to high society. Alice's husband was poor and his lack of income motivated Alice to have affairs with rich men so that she and her husband could keep up with London society. Alice's affairs were conducted with her husband's knowledge; he once said of her: "I do not mind what she does as long as she comes back to me in the end."

Apart from her beauty, Alice was well known for being kind, sunny and discreet. This last trait won her many admirers and brought her to the attention of the Prince of Whales, soon to be King Edward II. The King took Alice as his mistress and she stayed the royal mistress until his death in 1910.

The Intrigue of Alice

Alice Keppel was considered a beauty with her alabaster skin, chestnut hair, blue eyes, small waist and large bosom. Her kindness and charm always turned the King's melancholy moods into sunny ones.

Her elder daughter wrote "she not only had a gift of happiness but she excelled in making others happy, she resembled a Christmas tree laden with presents for everyone"

Buttermilk Mask for Alabaster Skin

Pat Buttermilk on your face with fingertips or cotton pad. Let dry for ten to fifteen minutes. Rinse with tepid water. The Buttermilk mask can also be used on the neck, shoulders, arms and bosom.

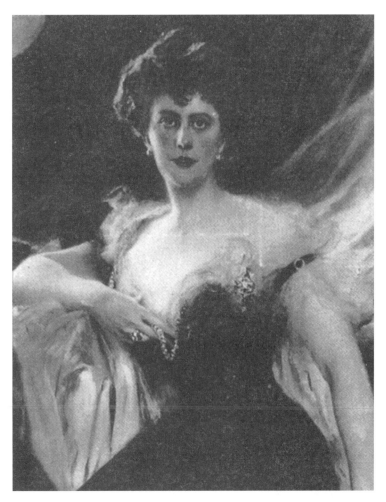

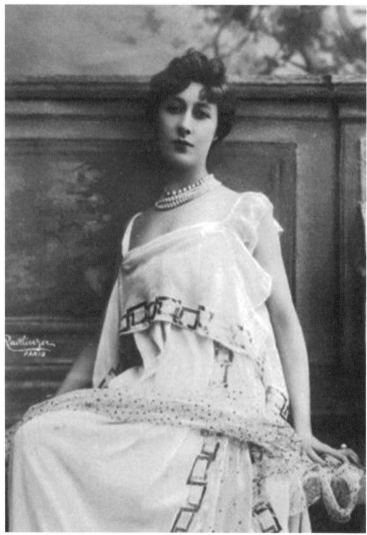

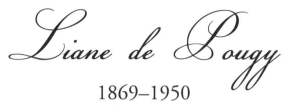

Liane de Pougy

1869–1950

Born: La Flèche, Sarthe, France
Birth Name: Anne Marie Chassaigne

"Father, except for murder and robbery – I've done everything."
~ Liane de Pougy

Who was Liane de Pougy?
Liane de Pougy was a famed and contemporary Parisian courtesan. Like La Belle Otero, Liane was a dancer at the Folies Bergères, but only occasionally so. The two of them battled back and forth between lovers and fame. Liane was famous and continually sought after by wealthy men. She made a point to know about literature and art, but not too much to "be boring." In the midst of her notoriety, she had a lesbian affair with writer Natalie Clifford Barney which added to her erotic reputation.

The Intrigue of Liane

Liane was a slender brunette who is purported to have started each day with an enema to keep "her skin clear and her breath sweet." She had servants that helped administer the enema and spent the rest of her mornings lounging in bed. During the time, it was believed that regular enemas could rid the body of excess toxins that would otherwise shorten the life span.

Liane's Salt Water Enema

It is suggested that Liane de Pougy had an enema every morning. An enema is the injection of liquid into the anus to cleanse the colon. Given that she had an enema every morning, she most likely had a salt water enema which would have been more gentle for daily use since it neither removes electrolytes from the body nor draws water into the colon.

To perform a salt water enema, first start with the solution. Mix 1 teaspoon salt (non iodized) for every pint of warm, filtered water. Administer the enema using an enema kit and directions and retain as long as possible (up to 40 minutes) then use the rest room.

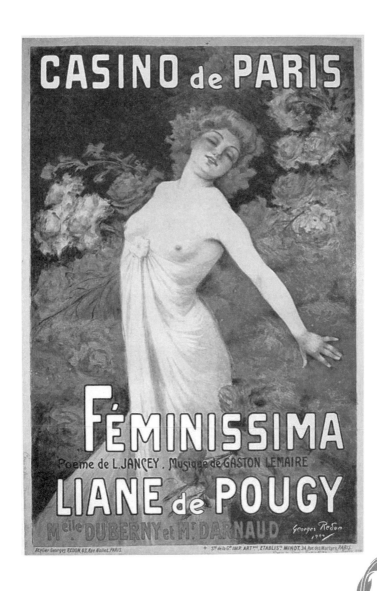

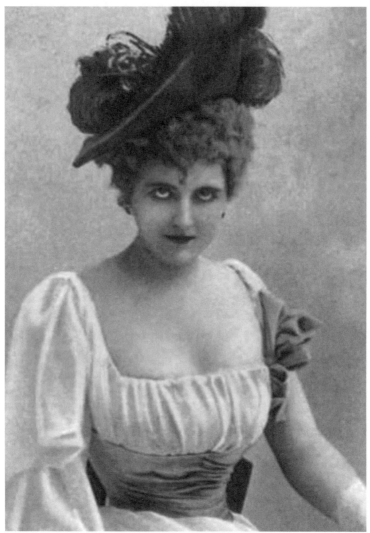

Clara Ward,
Princesse de
Caraman-Chimay

1873–1916
Born: Detroit, Michigan

Who was Clara Ward?

Clara Ward was born to a wealthy family in Michigan. Her
father was an iron and steel magnate and the first ever
millionaire in Michigan. Clara came to the public's
attention when a visiting Belgian prince and diplomat
proposed marriage to her. The Belgian prince was twice her
age and poor, but with marriage to him, she was awarded
the title of Princess. After having two children with her
prince, Clara left the prince and eloped with a Hungarian
Gypsy musician with whom she had fallen madly in love.
Her new husband played violin while Clara gave her "poses
plastiques," performance.

She would often wear flesh-colored skin tight body stockings when performing. The audience loved it. Artists and photographers paid her to have private sittings. Her beauty was deemed so "disturbing" by Kaiser Wilhelm II, that he forbade the publication or display of her photograph in the German Empire. The marriage between Clara and the Hungarian didn't last long. Clara performed on stage at the Folies Bergères and Moulin Rouge.

The Intrigue of Clara

Clara was beautiful for her time, tall, blonde and very voluptuous. It is said she was shaped like a goddess, but by today's standards was most likely overweight. What added to her intrigue was that she was unpredictable to the public. Public perception and opinion went wild with this wealthy daughter turned princess, turned gypsy traveler, turned French can-can girl.

Rinse for Clara's Fine Golden Hair

Mix equal quantities of hydrogen peroxide and warm water and use as a final rinse.
Warning: Using hydrogen peroxide on your hair can give it an orange, brassy color. This technique is best used by people with naturally light hair.

Lemon Juice Lightener

Squeeze the juice of one half lemon into a pint of water and use as a final rinse.

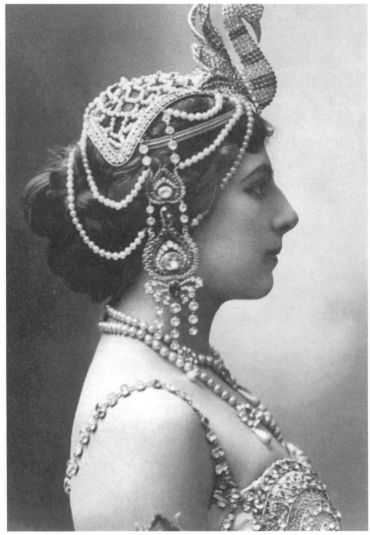

Mata Hari

1876–1917
Born: Leeuwarden, Netherlands
Birth Name: Margaretha Geertruida "M'greet"
Zelle MacLeod

Who Was Mata Hari?
"Mata Hari" was the eccentric name used by Margaretha MacLeod, a Dutch exotic dancer and courtesan. Mata Hari is most famous for being a convicted spy on the side of Germany during WW I. Mata Hari was found guilty of espionage and was executed by firing squad. It is said that on the eve of her execution, she asked for a milk bath.

The Intrigue of Mata Hari
The persona that Margaretha created was one of a "woman from the Far East...laden with perfume and jewels," an exotic Javanese dancer. She would dance and whirl with colorful veils, discarding them like a burlesque dancer to impart and create a sense of naughtiness. She was gorgeous and born blonde, but dyed her hair blue-black to further make people believe that she was from the "Orient."

Mata Hari's Blue-Black Hair Dye of the Orient

Period sources mention that Mata Hari was born with blonde hair, but dyed her hair blue-black. A popular way to dye the hair blue-black during the time period was to do a multi-step dye process using henna and indigo. The process was as follows. Wash the hair and apply a paste of henna (made from powdered henna and lukewarm water). Leave the paste on for an hour, then rinse off with lukewarm water. Let the hair dry slightly. Make a similar paste from powdered indigo (black henna) and water. Wait until the green powder turns black from the added water. Apply that to the hair and leave on for another hour, then rinse with lukewarm water. The hairs which were colored orange-red by the henna, now have a greenish-black appearance, but by the oxidation of the indigo in a short time acquire an intensely blue-black color, which is extraordinarily durable.

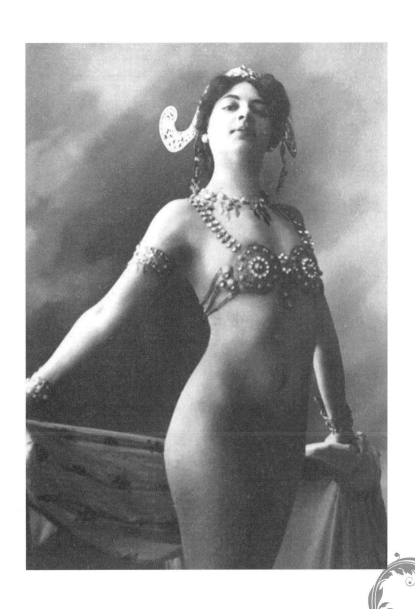

More Secrets

Wheat Bran Bath Water

Wrap 1-2 cups of dry bran in cloth, add to bath water. Used to beautify and soften the skin.

Orange Flower Water Bath

Add 1 cup orange flower water and 3 to 4 ounces of glycerin to bath water. Imparts skin with a delicacy and a delightful sensation of softness.

Heavy Cream

Applied to skin and used to prevent chapped hands, lips, and nipples.

Court Skin Whitening Wash

Infuse wheat-bran, well sifted, for four hours in white wine vinegar; add to it 5 egg yolks and 2 grains ambergris or musk; and distill the whole. It should be carefully corked for 12 to 15 days, when it will be fit for use.

They would apply it every time they made their toilet. It would give a polished whiteness to the neck and arms and a fine luster to the skin. Was also applied in the evening and left on overnight and rinsed off in the morning.

Perfumed Skin Wash

Combine 1 quart jasmine flower water and 1 quart orange flower water. To this can be added a scruple of both musk and ambergris.

Madam Vestris' Anti-Wrinkle Paste & Mask

Boil the whites of 4 eggs in a little rose water, half and ounce of alum, and half and ounce of sweet almond oil. Heat the whole together until it becomes the consistency of paste.

Spread the paste on silk or muslin and leave on skin overnight.

Benzoin Skin Wash (from the Court of Charles II)

Take a small piece of gum benzoin and boil it in spirits of wine until it becomes a rich tincture. Fifteen drops of this poured into a glass of water will produce a milky mixture. Apply to the skin. If left on the skin to dry it will render the skin clear and beautiful.

White Brandy Face Wash

Mix two parts white brandy with one part rose water and wash the face with it night and morning. Leaves the skin naturally soft and flexible.

Denmark Lotion

Take equal parts of the seeds of melon, pumpkin, gourd and cucumber, and grind until powdered. Add to this heavy cream to dilute the flour and then some milk to reduce the whole to a thin paste. Add a grain of musk and a few drops of oil of lemon. Anoint the face with this, leave on 20 to 30 minutes, and wash off with warm water. It gives a remarkable purity and brightness to the skin.

Pimpernel Water Face Wash

Used for whitening the complexion. Steep the plant in pure rainwater. Use as a wash.

French Milk of Roses

3 drams almond paste
½ pint rose water
½ fluid ounce tincture of benzoin
Mix almond paste and benzoin together and gradually add
rosewater while constantly stirring.

For Beautiful White Hands

Sleep with white kid gloves on your hands.

Dry Hand Lotion

3 ounces lemon juice
3 ounces white wine vinegar
½ pint white brandy

Macassar Hair Oil
(used by Ninon de l'Enclos)

Used as a hair conditioner to groom and style the hair.
1 pint castor oil or almond oil that has been reddened with
alkanet root (achieved by steeping 2 or 3 drams of root in
each pint of oil for 2 to 3 days)
½ pint alcohol
½ fluid drams oil of nutmeg
15 drops of rosemary oil
15 drops oregano oil
10 drops Neroli oil
4 or 5 drops essence of musk
20 grains otto of roses
Mix and agitate for some time. In a week decant or separate
the clear portion from the rest, if necessary. Should the
ingredients not mix thoroughly when shaken, cork and
place bottle in a bit of warm water and then cool again.

Honey Water Hair Cleanser

1 drams essence of ambergris
1 drams essence of musk
2 drams essence of bergamot
15 drops oil of cloves
4 ounces orange flower water
5 ounces wine
4 ounces distilled water
Mix all ingredients together and let sit for about 14 days.
Then filter and bottle for use.

Hair Removal

Spread on a piece of leather equal parts of galbanum and
pitch plaster, and lay it on the hairs as smoothly as possible.
After letting it remain on the hairs about 3 minutes pull it
off suddenly, taking the hair out by the roots.

Blackhead Wash

1 ounce liquor of potassa
2 ounces cologne
4 ounces white brandy
Apply a little of the above mixture to offending spots.

Anti-Freckle Wash

In the morning wash the skin with a combination of elder flower water and rose water.

Rice Water Skin Wash

Boil 1 cup of rice in four cups of water. Strain, keeping the liquid. Let liquid cool and use as a facial rinse.

Pomade de Seville

Mix equal parts lemon juice and whites of eggs. Beat
together and set over low heat and stir with a wooden spoon
until it acquires the consistency of a soft pomade. Used after
washing the face with rice water wash. It is said to remove
freckles and five a fine luster to the skin.

Anti-Wrinkle Facial Steam

In a hot pan over low heat, add powdered myrrh. Cover
head with a handkerchief and let face steam. Discontinue
if you feel any ill effect. Can also add a mouthful of white
wine to the hot myrrh and let smoke enter pours.

Cocoa Butter Lip Salve

Melt together equal parts cocoa butter, almond oil, and
white wax or beeswax. Remove from heat and stir until
nearly cold. Used as an emollient skin-cosmetic,
particularly for chapped lips, hands, etc.

Rouges

Rouge (red colorant) was used to "enhance" the complexion. It was used on the cheeks and lips. Rouge was created using many pigments, some toxic, some less so. Below are a few less-toxic/non-toxic pigments that were used and some recipes. It was usually applied with a camel hair pencil, hare's foot, or small powder puff. It was also used in the form of pomade, tinctured crepe (rouge crepons) and sometimes in a solution (liquid rouge). Used as rouge pigments:

-- Cochineal (carmine)
-- Bastard saffron
-- Safflower
-- Sandalwood
-- Madder Root
-- Alkanet Root
-- Red Ochre

Pigments can be used as...
-- a powder when mixed with rice powder or orris root.
-- an oil when mixed with almond oil or olive oil.
-- a liquid when mixed with vinegar, brandy or wine.

Carmine Rouge Powder

4 ounces rice powder
2 drams almond oil
1 ounce carmine

Liquid Rouge

Carmine can be diluted with rose water or alcohol and used as liquid rouge.

Vinegar Rouge

Take red sandalwood finely ground, and strong vinegar twice distilled, then put into it as much sandalwood as possible and let it simmer over low heat. Add a little powdered alum and you shall have "a very perfect red."

Wine Rouge

Take Brazil wood and rock alum; pound and add them to a bottle of red wine, and boil it till it is reduced to one fourth part. To use this, dip a piece of cotton wool into it, and rub the cheeks.

Sandalwood Rouge Oil

Take half an ounce of red sandalwood, half an ounce of cloves, and five ounces of sweet almonds. Pound the whole together. Upon this paste pour two ounces of white wine, and an ounce and a half of rose water. Let the whole be stirred up well together. In about eight or nine days, strain this paste and a very good red oil will be obtained.

Rouge Crepon / Spanish Wool (Hidden Alkanet Root Rouge)

Sometimes using paints was severely looked down upon. Women would need to hide or conceal their toilet items. Fabrics and items could be "dyed" ahead of time and used when needed to apply rouge and colorant. Alkanet root strikes a beautiful red when mixed with oils or pomatums. A scarlet or rose-colored ribbon, wetted with water or brandy, gives the cheeks if rubbed with it a beautiful bloom, that can scarcely be distinguished from the natural color. Some only use a cotton wool or sponge dyed with a colorant, which tinges the cheeks of a fine carnation color.

Violet Powder (face, hair, and dusting powder)

Finely powdered rice starch or potato starch scented with powdered orris root.

Facial Powders for Pale Looking Skin

Just as rouges, many of the powders were created using toxic ingredients. Below are a few non-toxic powders that were used.

The following were used as facial powders:
-- Pearl powder. This is made from real pearls.
-- Faux Pearl Powder. Made of bismuth, but this was toxic.
-- Rice powder
-- Potato powder
-- Magnesium carbonate

For a translucent dusting, apply powder with a dry cosmetic brush over skin to which has been applied moisturizer or foundation. Loose powder needs something to "stick" to. Dip cosmetic brush into powder, and then tap brush on tissue paper to remove extra powder. Lightly dust over the skin.

For more coverage, apply powder with a damp sponge (if no foundation) or dry sponge (if foundation has been applied). Press the powder onto the skin. Buff with stiff, dry cosmetic brush.

A final quote

"*Many of them live in palaces fit for great princes, and when you enter one of them you seem to be approaching the paradise of Venus. Their rooms are brilliantly lighted and furnished; the walls hung with rich tapestries and stamped leather...*

The courtesan comes forward to meet you dressed like a queen or the Goddess of Love....Her face is wonderfully beautiful; the lily and the rose wage war on her cheeks; her hair is raised in two points on her head so as to look almost like a pyramid. Her ornaments are so splendid that she at once arouses and captivates your senses, and causes you to lose your wits. You will find her like a second Cleopatra, covered with gold, chains, pearls, rings, diamonds, and other precious stones, with pendants of infinite value in her ears. Her skirt is of damask, with a fine fringe of gold or else gold lace; the chemise of red taffeta with gold fringes, stockings of red silk; her dress and her whole person perfumed so as to attract you more.

Moreover she will try and fascinate you by drawing sweet melodies from the lute, which she can play like a professor, or else by the tones of her voice, which go straight to your heart. You will find in her (if she is a person of distinction) an elegant conversationalist, and if she does not captivate you by the other arts I have named, she will try the charms of speech. To complete her sorceries she will subject you to the grandest temptation of all by taking you into her room. Here you will find painted furniture and number-less beautiful objects, a white canopy wrought with needle work, a silk coverlid sewn with gold thread, all breathing most delicious perfumes. Amid all these objects of luxury she will show you only one, and that an object which suggests mortification rather than delight; by her bed – a strange thing to find – a picture of the Madonna"

~ Coryat, Crudities, II

Index

A

B

C

Other Titles From Streamline Press

Art Deco Hair
Hairstyles from the 1920s & 1930s

1940s Hairstyles

1950s Hairstyles
Hairstyles from the Atomic Age of Cool

Vintage Beauty
Your Guide to Classic Hollywood Make-at-Home Beauty Treatments

Risque Beauty
Beauty Secrets of History's Most Notorious Courtesans

Vintage Wedding
Simple Ideas for Creating a Romantic Vintage Wedding

Rosie's Riveting Recipes
Cooking, Cocktails, and Kitchen Tips from 1940s America

Vintage Candy
An Essential Guide to Retro & Classic Candymaking

Amazing Science Play for Toddlers
Hands-On Science Activities for Bright & Gifted Kids

Huck Finn's Outdoor Adventure Guidebook
Activities & Projects Inspired by
The Adventures of Huckleberry Finn

For more information on books from Streamline Press,
please visit:
www.StreamlinePressShop.com
or visit us on Facebook at facebook.com/StreamlinePress